Dinner Menu for a Family Doc:

Narrative Medicine 'to-go'

It all started at dinner time, 'off-duty' when she really caught my attention. I had to listen carefully because here was something to learn! She told me about her experience with chronic pain and the details of what helped her out of a downward spiral. I can still hear her speaking:

"A turning point for me was an eight week yoga practice program that I attended. I didn't feel like a patient. I didn't have to tell my story. I could simply go there and get help. I was just a normal person."

1

"*I was encouraged to become active, to make the intangible tangible and develop solutions.*"

I felt like her experience gave the concept of 'empowerment' meaning.

She *didn't feel like a patient* and *was required to become active* and *felt in control.*

What this meant for her was hard to put into words, but she attempted to describe it in the following way:

Dr Fabian Schwarz - Dinner Menu for a Family Doc: Narrative Medicine 'to-go'

"It's much more than a choice to be proactive. First I went through the motions of being proactive (exercises and stretches, tried a gym membership and many types of therapies) but I didn't know how to make my thoughts proactive or accept my current weaknesses and limitations.

There were tools that had to be learnt, which can be different for each individual: to set goals or intentions for yourself, decide where to invest your energy and so on."

Dr Fabian Schwarz - Dinner Menu for a Family Doc: Narrative Medicine 'to-go'

I sense that my friend has many more insights to share. She continues to remind me of the kind of help she got out of her yoga practice:

"It was help that I could take with me – for example: I became aware of feeling anxious when driving. I noticed my breathing became shallow and fast. Then pain kicked in. I made the connection - just because I felt stressed didn't mean that I needed to have pain and vice versa. I could break the cycle."

Dr Fabian Schwarz - Dinner Menu for a Family Doc: Narrative Medicine 'to-go'

I felt like something just clicked, a switch, light dawned. It's not exactly a new scientific discovery but applied knowledge, customized to an individual's life situation. It is narrative based medicine in action. I just witnessed a powerful personal description of how self-awareness and reflection, combined with physical strategies such as breathing techniques, can help untangle situations and overcome some of the complexities of pain. Isn't she describing some of the aspects of empowerment?

The lesson didn't end there.

Dr Fabian Schwarz - Dinner Menu for a Family Doc: Narrative Medicine 'to-go'

My dinner guest continued:

"I had healthcare provider fatigue. I was so tired of running to appointments. I was sick of telling my story over and over again to different healthcare providers who gave different recommendations. Nothing really seemed to work. I was so passive. I did what I was told, but it didn't work. When you are in a desperate stage you do anything that you are told. I was hoping for help. But I felt like a victim to the healthcare and insurance systems. I felt like I had no control over my life."

Dr Fabian Schwarz - Dinner Menu for a Family Doc: Narrative Medicine 'to-go'

"I scheduled my life around appointments but there was nobody who really coordinated my care. There wasn't much consistency either. It was emotionally draining."

It was coming together. It started to make sense. It wasn't the first time I heard an encounter like that. However, how much has it influenced my practice as family physician?

Dr Fabian Schwarz - Dinner Menu for a Family Doc: Narrative Medicine 'to-go'

I felt like she was describing the role I am supposed to have as a family physician.

I have the opportunity to get to know the people who come to me.

I can make an effort to get more than just a snapshot in time.

I am supposed to be more than an executor of evidence-based-medicine with the latest medication and medical knowledge.

Here I was listening to an individual's story emphasizing components of the art of medicine:

Dr Fabian Schwarz - Dinner Menu for a Family Doc: Narrative Medicine 'to-go'

Applying knowledge to the individuals' circumstances and allowing an individual to be an individual human being and helping them to help themselves as well, not just matching or categorizing a case with a diagnosis.

It was at dessert time that my friend mentioned the concept of the half-way-house:

"I wish I could create a place where people can go to get help. Something like a half-way house, where there is the right balance of assistance and challenge, of support and stimulation, of real life and protection to prepare for the stressors and battles of daily life."

Dr Fabian Schwarz - Dinner Menu for a Family Doc: Narrative Medicine 'to-go'

First I felt like she was describing the concept of

rehab from a truly holistic point of view.

But it's seems more than that:

It's the place between a healthcare facility and a

patient's private home.

It's where people are allowed to find a refuge,

support and encouragement to take charge of their

life.

Exercise and healthy diets are naturally part of that.

But it goes far beyond the physical and

psychological aspects that are usually addressed.

"If you are dependent on something you want to become independent. The half-way-house is about enabling and creating an environment where there is a positive addiction – an addiction to improvement and personal development. So that people can succeed in their real-life circumstances."

Again I'm reminded of the concept of empowerment and wonder about the role I have as a family physician.

Isn't there something more I can do to create this environment in my practice?

Dr Fabian Schwarz - Dinner Menu for a Family Doc: Narrative Medicine 'to-go'

"I wish I could act as a peer consultant, to allow people with similar circumstances to navigate their way and recover more quickly. People have to stand up for themselves and take control, take responsibility and become proactive."

That was intriguing: *A peer consultant.*

That's a way towards creating a half-way-house in my own clinical practice.

Dr Fabian Schwarz - Dinner Menu for a Family Doc: Narrative Medicine 'to-go'

NBM+EBM = family physician engaging with peer consultants to help an individual in need (Evidence based medicine from randomized-controlled-trials, meets consumer reality, narrative based medicine, also termed NBM.)

Dinner was over.

I was subject to narrative medicine in practice.

I learnt.

I listened to my friend's journey through the land of chronic pain:

She started off as a passive passenger on the healthcare system train, faithfully attending appointment by appointment and experiencing 'healthcare provider fatigue'.

The scenery didn't change and she became worn out by recounting her story over and over again, reliving the trauma.

Dr Fabian Schwarz - Dinner Menu for a Family Doc: Narrative Medicine 'to-go'

There were very dark nights. The taste of joy was exotic, it was longed for. She navigated her way through the healthcare system.

Ultimately she came to a turning point, exiting the loop of the roller coaster.

She became more than a patient.

She started to be actively involved in her own journey, making sense of things she had seen and experienced, gradual improvement set in, thanks to very hard and ongoing work.

This work resulted in her learning to get to know herself, to overcome guilt and dependency.

Of course she had help from friends and family, but what enabled her to break through was an *active treatment approach* and her faith in God.

She still has a way to go, her journey isn't over, and many thoughts may still threaten her freedom. But she feels liberated and has found herself again.

Dr Fabian Schwarz - Dinner Menu for a Family Doc: Narrative Medicine 'to-go'

That's one big ongoing success story, which prompts me to engage people like her as *peer consultants* in my clinical practice. It's an attempt at creating the likes of a half-way-house. Because in our current model of care there is a big gap, which my friend describes as follows:

...it's a fact that practitioners only see me for the duration of my appointment and there is no possible way that they can see how I manage or cope with my daily circumstances...

There is much more to be said about *her experience* and what it means to *be empowered* and what *an active treatment approach* consists of.

There is a *need for people like my friend* to act as *peer consultants*.

Their role would be to fill parts of the gap created in a healthcare system; they would be in the position to focus on *the individual* and *how they manage their daily/practical circumstances* in a manner that only an insider can (one who has been there and can appreciate and then assist through first-hand knowledge/experience).

Dr Fabian Schwarz - Dinner Menu for a Family Doc: Narrative Medicine 'to-go'

Who is best qualified to answer questions like:

- *What is normal?*

- *What can I expect?*

- *Is it only me who feels this way?*

- *How do you navigate your way through the healthcare system?*

- *Where and how can I get help (to help myself) without wasting money, energy and time?*

- *What helped you?*

Obviously there is so much more to be said!

But now I have to thank my friend for a very rich

learning experience:

hearing *parts of her story,*

learning about her idea of the *half-way-house* and

describing the *essence of* what a *peer consultant* could

do in primary healthcare to help others toward

empowerment has been an absolute privilege.

I hope she will write and publish her story and ideas

for the sake of others, to help them on their journey.

Dr Fabian Schwarz - Dinner Menu for a Family Doc: Narrative Medicine 'to-go'

Dr Fabian Schwarz - Dinner Menu for a Family Doc: Narrative Medicine 'to-go'

_____

_____

_____

_____

_____

_____

Dr Fabian Schwarz - Dinner Menu for a Family Doc: Narrative Medicine 'to-go'

Dr Fabian Schwarz - Dinner Menu for a Family Doc: Narrative Medicine 'to-go'

_____

_____

_____

_____

_____

_____

_____

_____

_____

_____

_____

_____

Dr Fabian Schwarz - Dinner Menu for a Family Doc: Narrative Medicine 'to-go'

Dr Fabian Schwarz - Dinner Menu for a Family Doc: Narrative Medicine 'to-go'

www.ingramcontent.com/pod-product-compliance
Lightning Source LLC
Chambersburg PA
CBHW070800180526
45168CB00004B/1698